Isometric Workouts for Older Adults

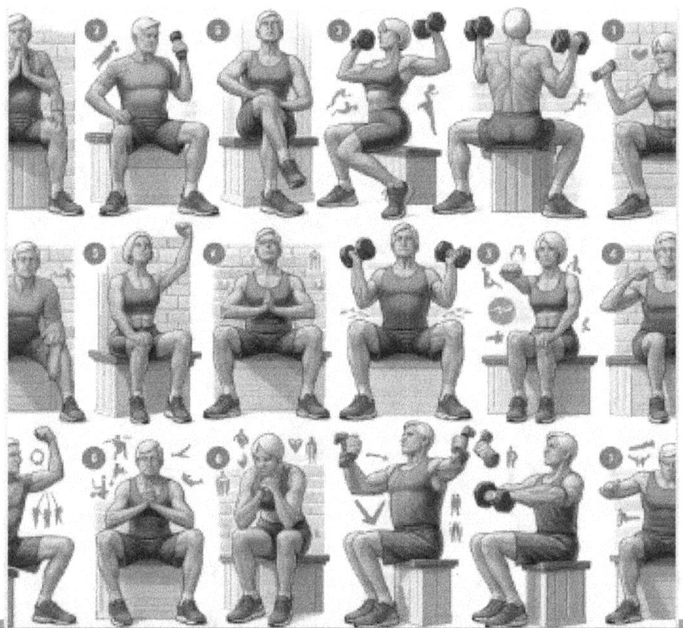

Unlocking Vitality and Wellness After 50 with Tailored Exercises for Age-Related Challenges

Troy Vhodes

Table of Contents

Introduction

In the twilight of our years, as the sun sets on one chapter of life, another beckons, promising vitality, strength, and boundless wellness. Welcome to "Isometric Workouts for Older Adults: Unlocking Vitality and Wellness After 50 with Tailored Exercises for Age-Related Challenges." Within these pages lies not just a fitness guide, but a testament to the transformative power of isometric exercises, a journey that transcends mere physicality to illuminate the path towards a life reinvigorated with vigor and purpose.

Picture this: It's a crisp morning, the gentle rustle of leaves harmonizing with the rhythmic beat of your heart as you embark on your isometric journey. You may be skeptical, perhaps even hesitant, but allow me to share a story, a story of triumph over adversity, of resilience, and of rediscovered strength.

Imagine a soul weary from the burdens of age, plagued by the relentless march of time. This was my reality, until isometric workouts breathed new life into my weary limbs. Through perseverance and dedication, I witnessed a metamorphosis, a transformation that defied age, defied expectations, and defied limitations.

But this journey is not just mine to tell. It belongs to countless others, each carving their path towards wellness, one isometric contraction at a time. From the spirited octogenarian reclaiming her independence to the seasoned veteran rediscovering the joy of movement, the stories are as diverse as they are inspiring.

Isometrics, with its simplicity and efficacy, offers more than just physical benefits, it offers hope. Hope for a future unencumbered by the shackles of age-related ailments. Hope for a life enriched by vitality, wellness, and unyielding resilience.

So, dear reader, I invite you to embark on this odyssey with me. Let us shatter preconceptions, defy expectations, and embrace the boundless potential that lies within. Let us unlock vitality and wellness after 50, not merely as a goal, but as a birthright, a testament to the indomitable spirit of the human endeavor.

Are you ready to seize the reins of your destiny? Are you ready to embrace a life redefined by strength, resilience, and boundless wellness? If so, then join me as we embark on this exhilarating journey together, a journey towards a future brimming with possibility. Let us take that first step, that first isometric contraction, and usher in a new era of vitality and wellness. The time is now. The journey begins.

Chapter 1
The Science Behind Isometric Exercises
Exploring the Benefits of Isometric Training for Seniors

Welcome to the foundation of our isometric journey! In this chapter, we'll delve into the fascinating world of isometric training and uncover the multitude of benefits it holds for seniors. But before we dive in, let's take a moment to appreciate the marvel of the human body and the incredible potential that lies within.

Imagine your body as a finely tuned instrument, capable of remarkable feats of strength and endurance. Now, picture isometric exercises as the conductor, orchestrating symphonies of movement and vitality within your muscles. It's a partnership rooted in science, where the principles of physiology and biomechanics converge to sculpt a stronger, more resilient you.

As we embark on this exploration, let's adopt an informal, conversational tone, imagine we're chatting over a cup of coffee, sharing insights and anecdotes that ignite the spark of curiosity within you. So grab a seat, settle in, and let's unlock the secrets of isometric training together.

Now, you might be wondering, what exactly are isometric exercises, and how do they differ from other forms of training?

Well, think of isometric exercises as the steady, unwavering foundation upon which your strength and stability are built. Unlike dynamic movements that involve joint motion, isometric exercises involve contracting your muscles without changing their length or joint angle. It's like pressing against an immovable object, feeling the tension build within your muscles as they work against resistance.

But why choose isometric training, you ask? Ah, that's where the magic lies! Let's explore the benefits:

1. Strengthens Muscles Without Joint Strain:

Isometric exercises provide a safe and effective way to build muscle strength without putting undue stress on your joints. By holding static positions, you can target specific muscle groups with precision, gradually increasing resistance as you grow stronger.

2. Enhances Joint Stability:

As we age, maintaining joint stability becomes increasingly important to prevent injuries and maintain mobility. Isometric exercises help improve joint stability by strengthening the surrounding muscles and ligaments, providing a solid foundation for movement.

3. Improves Posture and Balance:

Picture yourself standing tall and proud, your spine aligned, and your shoulders back, all thanks to the power of isometric exercises. By targeting the muscles responsible for posture and balance, isometric training can help you stand taller, move with greater ease, and reduce the risk of falls.

4. Boosts Functional Strength:

Whether you're lifting groceries, climbing stairs, or simply getting out of bed in the morning, everyday activities require strength and endurance. Isometric exercises mimic these functional movements, helping you build strength that translates seamlessly into your daily life.

So there you have it, the science behind isometric exercises laid bare. But our journey is just beginning! In the chapters ahead, we'll delve deeper into the world of isometric training, exploring different exercises, techniques, and strategies to help you unlock your full potential. So, strap in, stay curious, and let's embark on this exhilarating adventure together!

Understanding How Isometric Exercises Impact Aging Bodies

As we age, our bodies undergo a multitude of changes, from declines in muscle mass and bone density to alterations in joint flexibility and overall mobility. These age-related changes can significantly impact our ability to perform daily activities and maintain independence, leading to a decline in overall quality of life. However, amidst these challenges, isometric exercises emerge as a powerful tool to combat the effects of aging and promote vitality and wellness well into our later years.

To truly grasp the impact of isometric exercises on aging bodies, it's essential to delve into the physiological mechanisms at play. Let's break it down:

1. Muscle Strength and Mass:

One of the most noticeable changes that occur with aging is the gradual loss of muscle strength and mass, a phenomenon known as sarcopenia. This decline in muscle mass can lead to decreased mobility, increased risk of falls, and compromised functional independence. Isometric exercises offer a solution by providing a stimulus for muscle growth and strength development without the need for heavy weights or dynamic movements. By engaging in isometric contractions, seniors can target specific muscle groups and stimulate muscle hypertrophy, thus counteracting the effects of sarcopenia and preserving overall muscle function.

2. Bone Density:

Another significant concern for aging bodies is the loss of bone density, a condition known as osteoporosis, which increases the risk of fractures and skeletal fragility. Isometric exercises have been shown to promote bone health by exerting mechanical stress on the skeletal system, stimulating osteoblast activity, and enhancing bone mineral density. By incorporating weight-bearing isometric exercises such as wall sits or planks into their routine, seniors can effectively strengthen their bones, reduce the risk of fractures, and maintain skeletal integrity well into old age.

3. Joint Stability and Flexibility:

Aging is often accompanied by a decrease in joint flexibility and stability, leading to stiffness, discomfort, and impaired mobility. Isometric exercises play a crucial role in improving joint health by strengthening the surrounding muscles and stabilizing the joint structures. By holding static positions and engaging in isometric contractions, seniors can enhance joint stability, increase range of motion, and alleviate joint pain and stiffness. Additionally, isometric exercises promote proprioception, the body's awareness of its position in space, thus improving balance and coordination and reducing the risk of falls.

4. Metabolic Health:

Beyond its impact on musculoskeletal health, isometric exercise also exerts beneficial effects on metabolic health, particularly in older adults. Studies have shown that isometric exercises can improve insulin sensitivity, lower blood pressure, and reduce visceral fat accumulation, thus reducing the risk of metabolic disorders such as diabetes and cardiovascular disease. By incorporating isometric exercises into their regular routine, seniors can promote overall metabolic health and enhance their quality of life.

In essence, the impact of isometric exercises on aging bodies is multifaceted and far-reaching, addressing key physiological changes associated with advancing age. From preserving muscle mass and bone density to promoting joint stability and metabolic health, isometric exercises offer a holistic approach to aging gracefully and maintaining vitality and wellness well into our later years. By embracing the power of isometric training, seniors can reclaim their strength, mobility, and independence, enabling them to lead active, fulfilling lives for years to come.

Chapter 2
Getting Started: Preparing for Your Isometric Journey
Assessing Your Fitness Level and Setting Realistic Goals

Embarking on your isometric journey is an exciting endeavor, a chance to reclaim strength, vitality, and wellness in your later years. But before you dive headfirst into your workouts, it's crucial to lay a solid foundation by assessing your current fitness level and setting realistic goals tailored to your individual needs and capabilities.

Assessing Your Fitness Level:

Before you begin any new exercise program, it's essential to take stock of your current fitness level to determine your starting point. This assessment not only helps you understand your strengths and areas for improvement but also ensures that you embark on your isometric journey safely and effectively.

Here are some key components to consider when assessing your fitness level:

1. Strength:

Evaluate your current strength by performing basic exercises such as squats, push-ups, or wall sits. Take note of how many repetitions you can comfortably complete and the level of difficulty you experience.

2. Flexibility:

Assess your flexibility by performing simple stretches targeting major muscle groups such as the hamstrings, quadriceps, and shoulders. Pay attention to any areas of tightness or limited range of motion.

3. Balance and Stability:

Test your balance and stability by standing on one leg for a set amount of time or performing simple balance exercises such as standing heel-to-toe or marching in place. Note any difficulty maintaining balance or instability.

4. Endurance:

Evaluate your cardiovascular endurance by engaging in activities that elevate your heart rate, such as brisk walking or cycling. Pay attention to how long you can sustain the activity and your perceived level of exertion.

Setting Realistic Goals:

Once you've assessed your fitness level, it's time to set realistic and achievable goals that align with your desires and capabilities. Setting clear goals provides direction and motivation, guiding your isometric journey and helping you track progress along the way.

Here are some tips for setting realistic goals:

1. Be Specific:

Define your goals with clarity, specifying what you want to achieve and how you plan to do it. For example, instead of setting a vague goal like "get stronger," aim for a specific target such as "increase my wall sit time by 30 seconds."

2. Make Them Measurable:

Ensure that your goals are measurable so that you can track your progress over time. Use concrete metrics such as repetitions, time, or distance to quantify your achievements.

3. Set Attainable Targets:

Be realistic about what you can accomplish given your current fitness level and lifestyle. Set targets that challenge you without overwhelming you, allowing for steady progress and success.

4. Consider Your Motivation:

Reflect on what motivates you to embark on your isometric journey and tailor your goals accordingly. Whether it's improving overall health, increasing strength, or reducing pain, align your goals with your underlying motivations to stay focused and committed.

5. Break Them Down:

Break larger goals into smaller, more manageable milestones to prevent feeling overwhelmed and maintain momentum. Celebrate each achievement along the way, no matter how small, as it brings you closer to your ultimate objectives.

By assessing your fitness level and setting realistic goals, you lay the groundwork for a successful and fulfilling isometric journey. Armed with a clear understanding of where you stand and where you want to go, you can approach your workouts with confidence, determination, and a sense of purpose, unlocking the full potential of your body and embracing a future brimming with vitality and wellness.

Creating a Safe and Supportive Exercise Environment

When embarking on your isometric journey, creating a safe and supportive exercise environment is paramount to your success and well-being. By establishing a space that fosters comfort, confidence, and accessibility, you set the stage for a positive and fulfilling workout experience. Let's delve into how you can create such an environment:

1. Clear Space:

Start by ensuring you have ample space to perform your isometric exercises safely and comfortably. Clear away any clutter or obstacles that could pose a tripping hazard, and designate a designated workout area free from distractions.

2. Proper Equipment:

While isometric exercises typically require minimal equipment, ensure that you have any necessary props or aids readily available. This may include a sturdy chair for support, a yoga mat for cushioning, or resistance bands for added resistance.

3. Adequate Lighting and Ventilation:

Make sure your exercise space is well-lit and properly ventilated to promote safety and comfort during your workouts. Natural light and fresh air can invigorate your senses and enhance your overall workout experience.

4. Supportive Flooring:

Choose a flooring surface that provides adequate cushioning and support, particularly if you'll be performing exercises that involve kneeling or lying down. Consider using a yoga mat or exercise mat to protect your joints and prevent discomfort.

5. Temperature Control:

Maintain a comfortable temperature in your exercise space to prevent overheating or discomfort during your workouts. Adjust the thermostat as needed and consider using fans or opening windows to regulate airflow and maintain an optimal workout environment.

6. Proper Form and Technique:

Focus on maintaining proper form and technique throughout your workouts to prevent injuries and maximize effectiveness. Pay attention to alignment, breathing, and muscle engagement, and seek guidance from a qualified instructor if needed.

7. Hydration and Nutrition:

Stay hydrated and nourished before, during, and after your workouts to support optimal performance and recovery. Keep a water bottle nearby and fuel your body with nutritious foods that provide sustained energy and replenish essential nutrients.

8. Supportive Community:

Surround yourself with a supportive community of like-minded individuals who share your goals and values.

Whether it's joining a fitness class, enlisting the support of friends and family, or connecting with online communities, having a support system can boost motivation, accountability, and overall enjoyment of your workouts.

By creating a safe and supportive exercise environment, you empower yourself to embark on your isometric journey with confidence, enthusiasm, and peace of mind. With the right tools, mindset, and surroundings, you can unlock the full potential of your body and embrace a future filled with vitality, wellness, and boundless possibilities.

Chapter 3
Mastering the Basics: Essential Isometric Techniques
Learning the Fundamentals of Isometric Contractions

Isometric exercises serve as the cornerstone of your journey towards strength, vitality, and wellness. In this chapter, we'll delve into the fundamentals of isometric contractions, providing you with step-by-step explanations of essential exercises to help you master the basics and lay a solid foundation for your isometric journey.

1. Wall Sit:

- Stand with your back against a sturdy wall and your feet hip-width apart.
- Slowly slide down the wall until your knees are bent at a 90-degree angle, with your thighs parallel to the floor.
- Press your lower back into the wall and engage your core muscles to maintain stability.
- Hold this position for as long as you can, aiming to gradually increase your hold time with each session.
- Focus on breathing deeply and evenly throughout the exercise, keeping your chest lifted and shoulders relaxed.

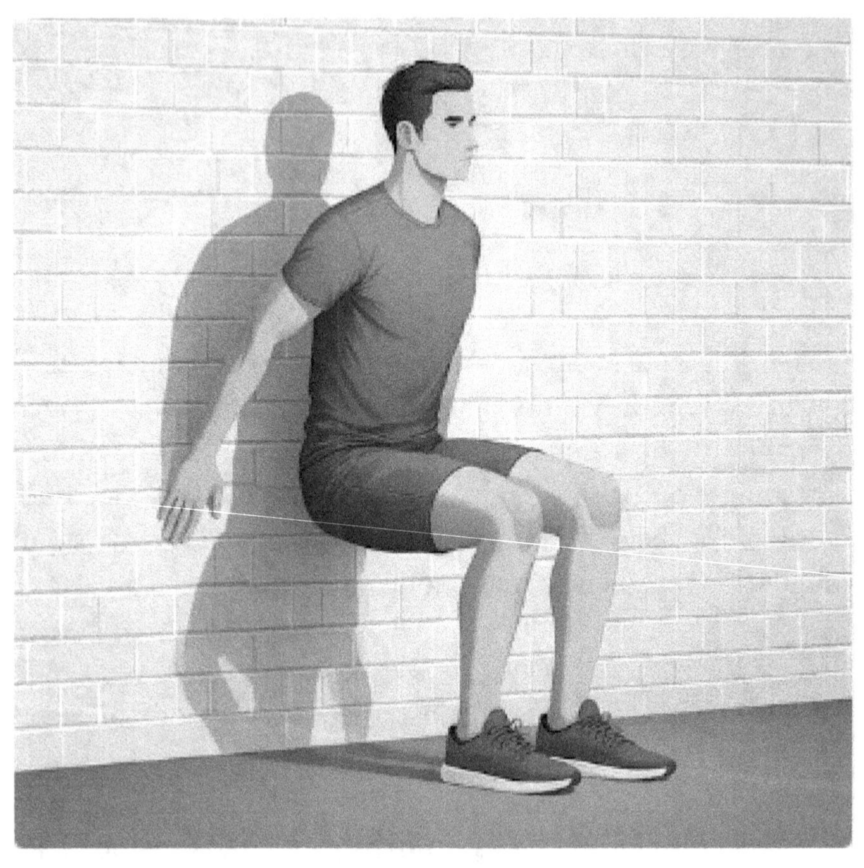

2. *Plank:*

- Begin in a push-up position with your hands shoulder-width apart and your body in a straight line from head to heels.
- Engage your core muscles and lower yourself onto your forearms, keeping your elbows directly beneath your shoulders.
- Maintain a neutral spine and avoid arching or rounding your back.
- Hold this position for as long as you can, aiming to keep your body in a straight line without sagging or lifting your hips.
- Focus on breathing steadily and maintaining tension throughout your entire body, from your shoulders to your toes.

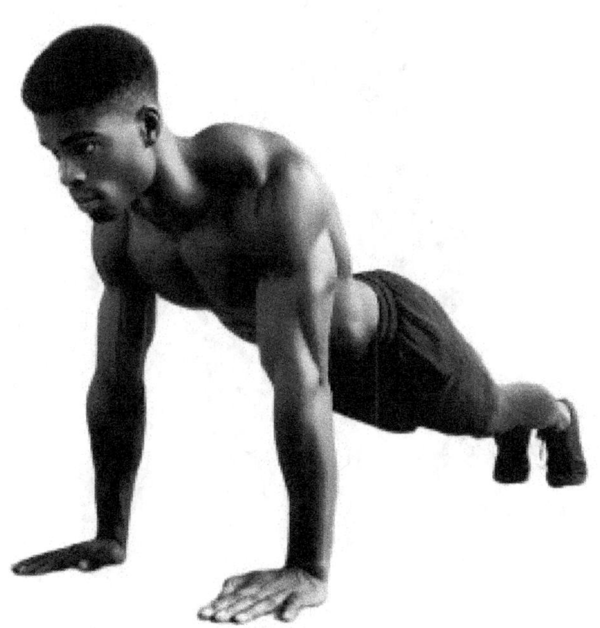

3. Static Lunge:

- Start by standing with your feet hip-width apart and take a large step backward with your right foot.
- Lower your body down into a lunge position, bending both knees to approximately 90-degree angles.
- Ensure that your front knee is aligned with your ankle and your back knee hovers just above the floor.
- Hold this position for a designated amount of time, then return to the starting position.
- Repeat the exercise on the opposite side, alternating legs with each repetition.

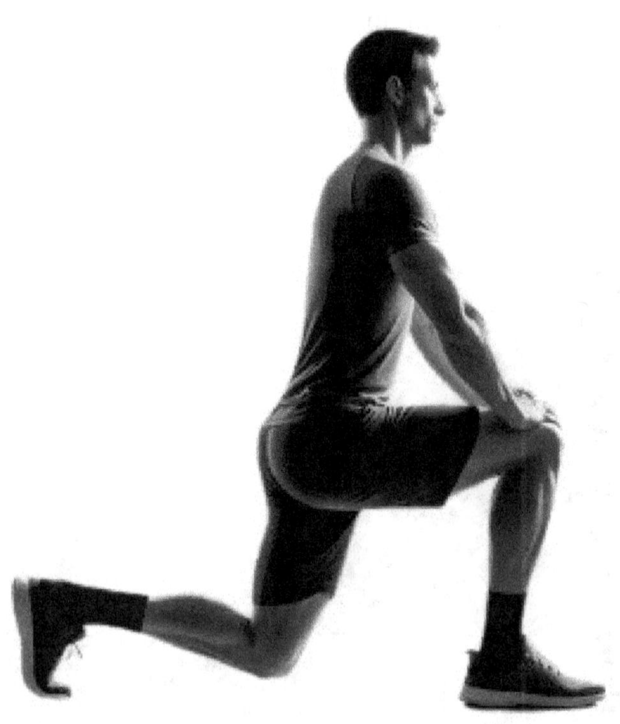

4. Chest Press Against Wall:

- Stand facing a sturdy wall with your feet hip-width apart and your arms extended in front of you at shoulder height.
- Press your palms firmly into the wall and engage your chest muscles as you push against the wall.
- Hold this position for a designated amount of time, focusing on maintaining tension in your chest muscles.
- Release the contraction and repeat for the desired number of repetitions.

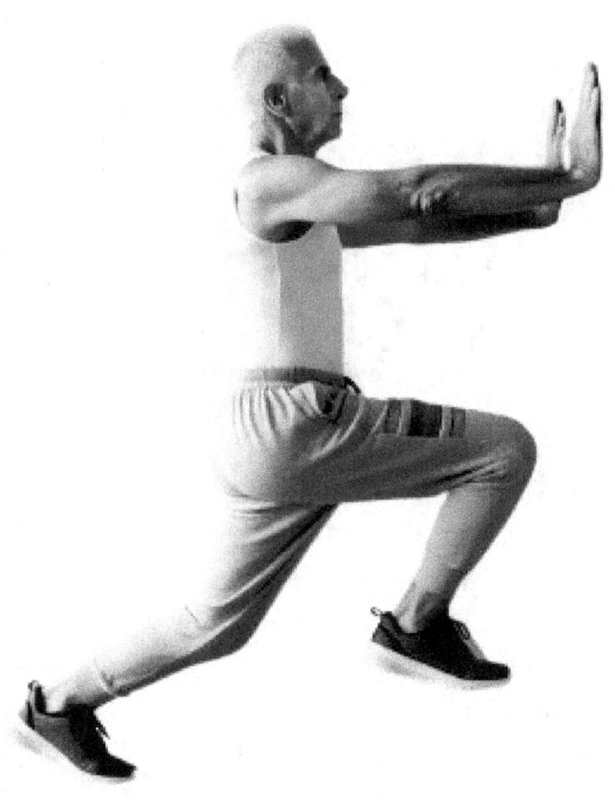

5. *Isometric Abdominal Crunch:*

- Lie on your back with your knees bent and your feet flat on the floor.
- Place your hands behind your head, with your elbows pointing outward.
- Lift your head, neck, and shoulders slightly off the floor, engaging your abdominal muscles.
- Hold this position for a designated amount of time, focusing on contracting your abdominal muscles.
- Release the contraction and repeat for the desired number of repetitions.

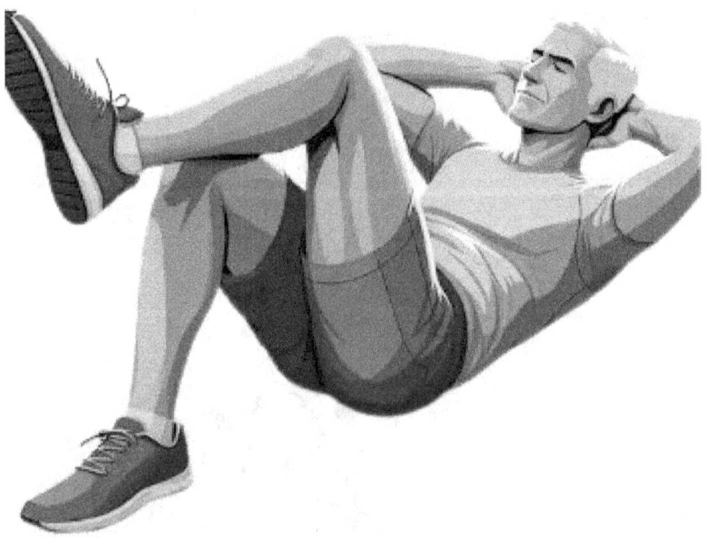

These essential isometric exercises form the building blocks of your workout routine, helping you develop strength, stability, and endurance from the ground up. By mastering the basics and incorporating these exercises into your regular workouts, you'll lay the groundwork for a stronger, healthier, and more resilient body, setting the stage for success on your isometric journey.

Practicing Proper Breathing and Form for Maximum Effectiveness

In the realm of isometric exercises, mastering proper breathing and form is essential for maximizing effectiveness and minimizing the risk of injury. In this section, we'll explore the importance of breathing and form in isometric training and provide practical tips for incorporating these elements into your workouts.

Breathing:

Proper breathing techniques play a crucial role in isometric exercises, helping you maintain stability, control, and focus throughout your workouts. Here's why mastering your breathing is so important:

1. Oxygenation:

Deep, controlled breathing ensures that your muscles receive an adequate supply of oxygen, enhancing endurance and performance during isometric contractions.

2. Core Engagement:

Proper breathing patterns can facilitate engagement of the core muscles, providing stability and support for the spine and pelvis during static holds.

3. Relaxation:

Conscious breathing promotes relaxation and reduces tension in the body, allowing you to achieve deeper levels of muscle relaxation and contraction.

To practice proper breathing during isometric exercises:

- Inhale deeply through your nose as you prepare to initiate the contraction.
- Exhale slowly and steadily through your mouth as you engage the target muscles and hold the contraction.
- Focus on maintaining a steady rhythm of breathing throughout each repetition, avoiding shallow or erratic breaths.
- Visualize your breath flowing smoothly and effortlessly, syncing with the movements of your body as you perform each exercise.

Form:

Form refers to the proper alignment, posture, and positioning of your body during isometric exercises. Maintaining correct form is crucial for targeting the intended muscle groups effectively and preventing strain or injury. Here's why form matters:

1. Muscle Activation:

Proper form ensures that the intended muscle groups are engaged and activated, maximizing the effectiveness of each exercise.

2. Joint Alignment:

Correct alignment reduces the risk of joint strain or injury, promoting safe and efficient movement patterns during isometric contractions.

3. Balance and Stability:

Good form promotes balance and stability, enabling you to maintain control and control over your body's position during static holds.

To practice proper form during isometric exercises:

- Align your body in a neutral position, with your spine straight, shoulders relaxed, and core engaged.
- Focus on maintaining proper alignment of your joints, ensuring that they are stacked vertically and in line with one another.
- Avoid excessive tension or arching in the spine, and be mindful of any areas of discomfort or strain.
- Use mirrors or visual cues to check your form periodically and make adjustments as needed.
- Start with lighter resistance or shorter hold times to ensure that you can maintain proper form throughout each repetition.

By prioritizing proper breathing and form in your isometric workouts, you can enhance the effectiveness of your exercises, reduce the risk of injury, and maximize the benefits of your training. With mindful attention to these fundamental elements, you'll lay a solid foundation for strength, stability, and vitality on your isometric journey.

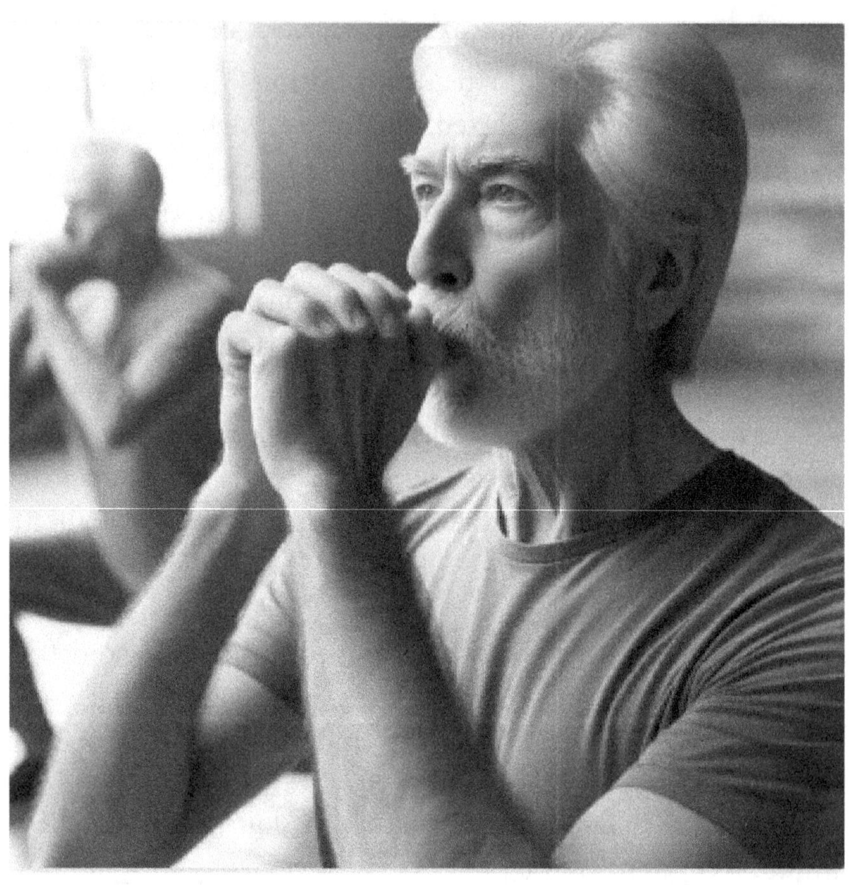

Chapter 4
Customizing Your Workout Routine
Tailoring Isometric Exercises to Address Common Age-Related Conditions

As we age, our bodies undergo changes that can present unique challenges to our fitness journey. However, with thoughtful customization, isometric exercises can be adapted to address common age-related conditions, promoting strength, mobility, and overall well-being. In this section, we'll explore how to tailor your workout routine to address specific concerns, providing step-by-step explanations for exercises targeting common age-related conditions.

1. Arthritis Relief and Joint Mobility:

Isometric Hand Grips:

- Sit or stand comfortably with your arms at your sides.
- Hold a soft ball or stress ball in one hand.
- Squeeze the ball firmly with your fingers and palm, holding the contraction for a few seconds.
- Release and repeat on the other hand.
- Aim for 10-15 repetitions on each hand, gradually increasing as tolerated.

Wall Push-Up:

- Stand facing a wall with your arms extended at shoulder height and your palms flat against the wall.
- Lean forward slightly, bending your elbows and bringing your chest towards the wall.
- Press into the wall, engaging your chest and arm muscles, and hold the contraction for a few seconds.
- Release and repeat for 10-15 repetitions, focusing on smooth, controlled movements.

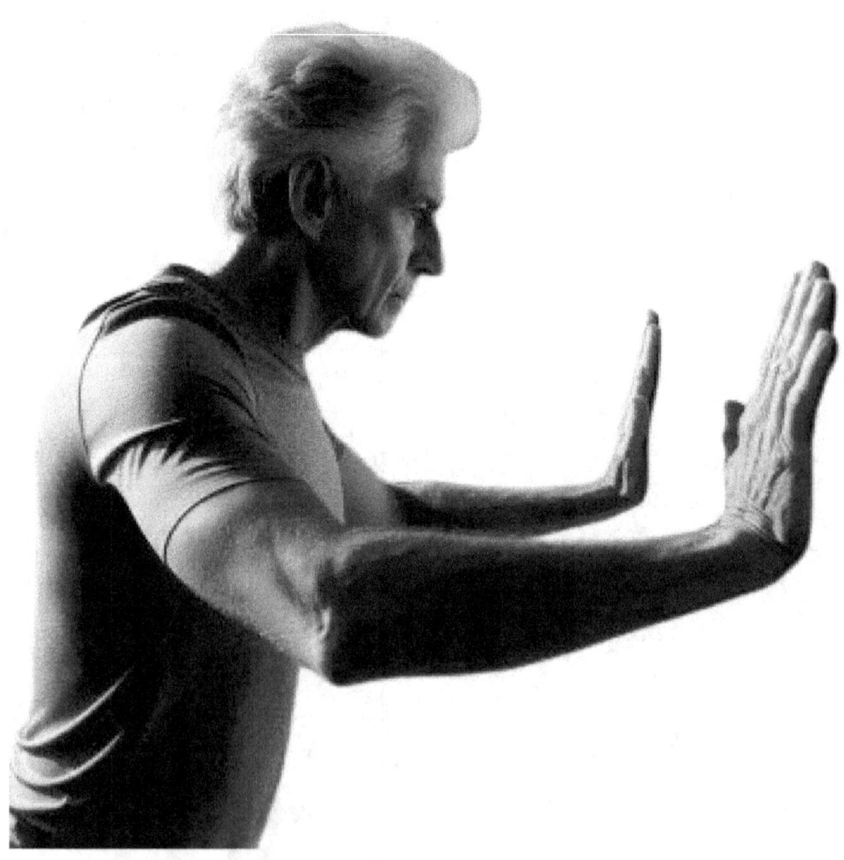

2. Strengthening Bones: Isometric Strategies for Osteoporosis Management:

Wall Sit with Calf Raises:
- Stand with your back against a sturdy wall and your feet hip-width apart.
- Lower into a wall sit position, bending your knees to a 90-degree angle and pressing your lower back into the wall.
- Hold the wall sit position and simultaneously lift your heels off the ground, rising onto the balls of your feet.
- Hold the calf raise position for a few seconds, then lower your heels back to the ground.
- Repeat the calf raises for 10-15 repetitions, focusing on maintaining proper form and alignment.

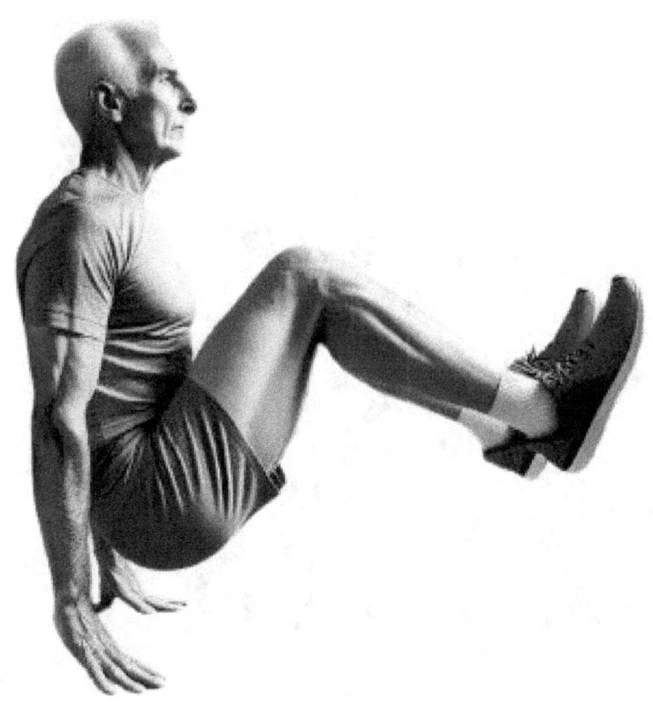

Isometric Abdominal Crunch with Leg Lift:

- Lie on your back with your knees bent and your feet flat on the floor.
- Place your hands behind your head, elbows pointing outward.
- Lift your head, neck, and shoulders slightly off the floor, engaging your abdominal muscles.
- Extend one leg straight out in front of you, hovering above the floor.
- Hold the isometric contraction for a few seconds, then return to the starting position and repeat on the opposite side.
- Aim for 10-15 repetitions on each leg, focusing on controlled movements and maintaining core stability.

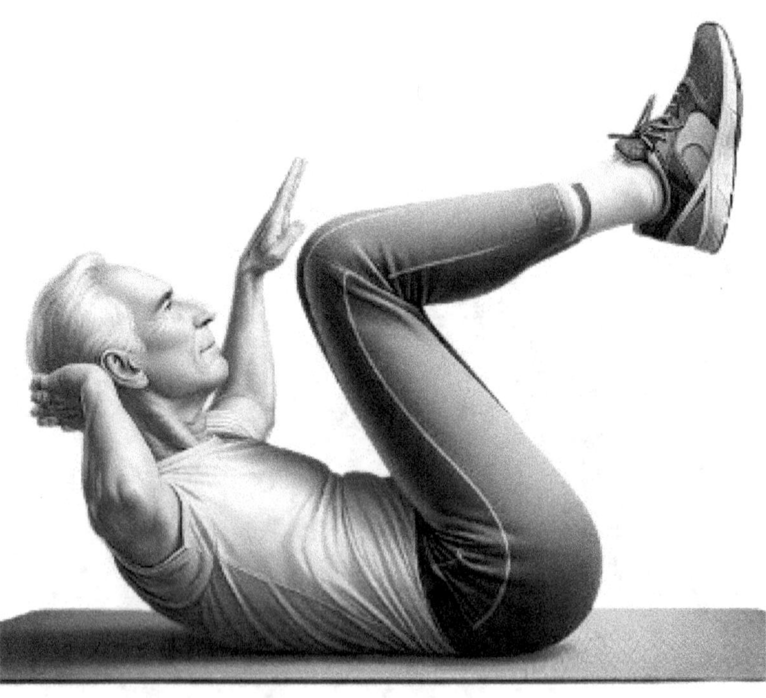

3. Enhancing Balance and Coordination:

Single-Leg Balance:

- Stand with your feet hip-width apart and your arms at your sides.
- Lift one foot off the ground and balance on the opposite leg.
- Engage your core muscles and focus on maintaining your balance for 20-30 seconds.
- Repeat on the opposite leg, aiming for 3-5 repetitions on each side.
- For added challenge, try closing your eyes or standing on a foam pad to further challenge your balance.

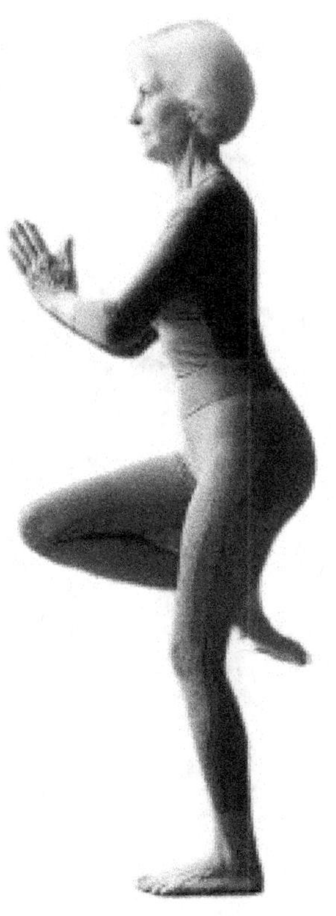

Isometric Side Leg Lift:

- Stand tall with your feet hip-width apart and your hands resting on a stable surface for support.
- Lift one leg out to the side, keeping it straight and parallel to the floor.
- Hold the lifted position for a few seconds, engaging your outer thigh and hip muscles.
- Lower your leg back to the starting position and repeat on the opposite side.
- Aim for 10-15 repetitions on each leg, focusing on controlled movements and maintaining proper alignment.

\

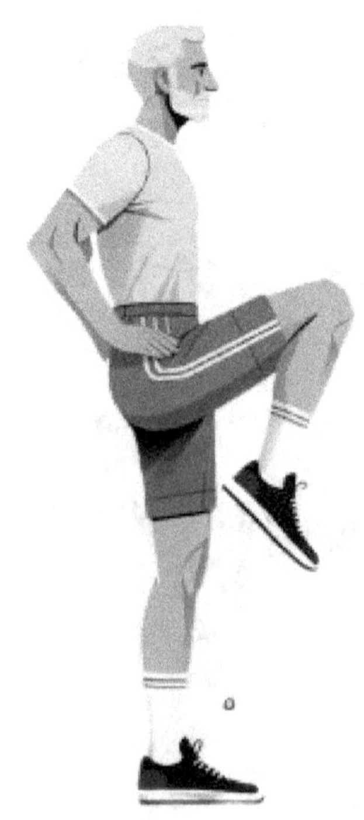

4. Improving Mobility and Flexibility:

Seated Leg Press:

- Sit on a sturdy chair with your feet flat on the floor and your knees bent at a 90-degree angle.
- Place your hands on the sides of the chair for support.
- Press your feet into the ground, engaging your thigh muscles, and lift one foot off the floor.
- Hold the lifted position for a few seconds, focusing on maintaining tension in your thigh muscles.
- Lower your foot back to the floor and repeat on the opposite side.
- Aim for 10-15 repetitions on each leg, gradually increasing as you build strength and mobility.

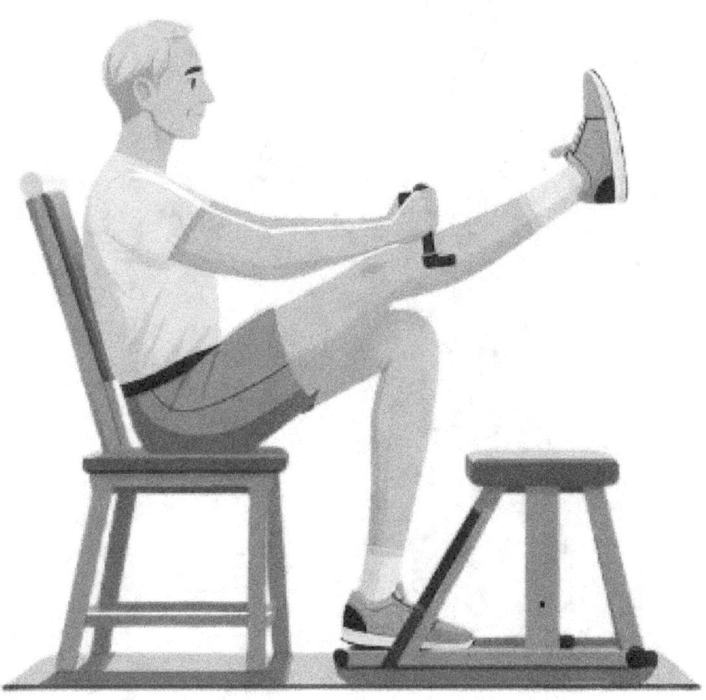

Isometric Chest Opener:

- Stand tall with your feet hip-width apart and your arms extended behind you.
- Clasp your hands together behind your back, palms facing inward.
- Gently squeeze your shoulder blades together and lift your hands away from your body, opening up your chest.
- Hold the contraction for a few seconds, focusing on stretching through your chest and shoulders.
- Release and repeat for 10-15 repetitions, breathing deeply and maintaining good posture throughout.

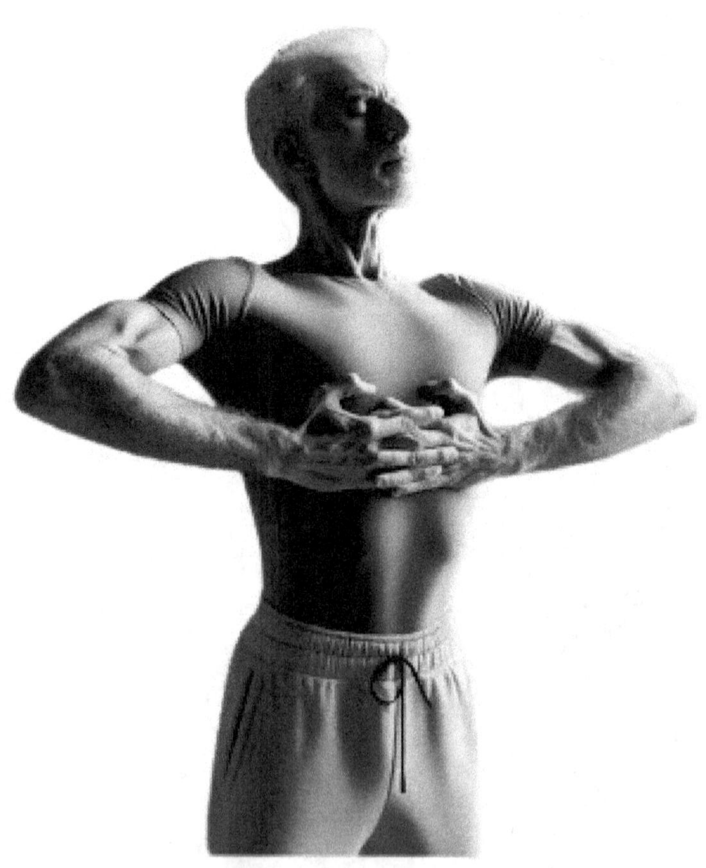

5. Managing Balance Disorders:

Chair Squat with Leg Lift:
- Begin by sitting on the edge of a sturdy chair with your feet flat on the floor.
- Stand up from the chair, pushing through your heels and engaging your thigh and glute muscles.
- Once standing, lift one leg off the ground and extend it forward, parallel to the floor.
- Hold the lifted position for a few seconds, focusing on maintaining balance and stability.
- Lower your leg back to the ground and return to the seated position.
- Repeat on the opposite leg for 10-15 repetitions, gradually increasing as your balance improves.

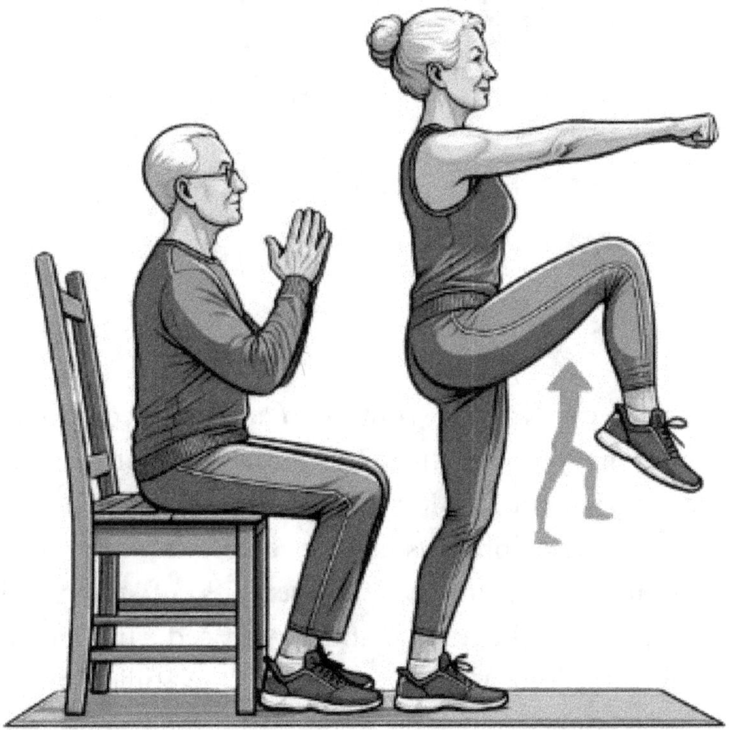

Isometric Toe Tap:

- Stand behind a stable surface such as a chair or countertop for support.
- Lift one foot slightly off the ground and tap your toe lightly in front of you.
- Hold the tapped position for a few seconds, focusing on maintaining stability through your standing leg.
- Return your foot to the starting position and repeat on the opposite side.
- Aim for 10-15 repetitions on each leg, focusing on controlled movements and maintaining balance throughout.

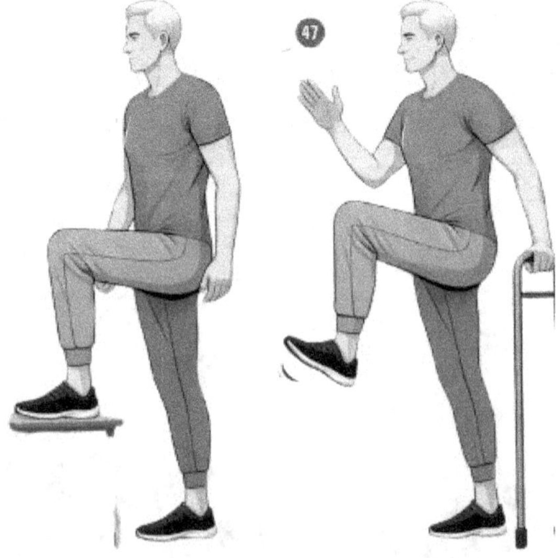

By customizing your workout routine to address specific age-related conditions, you can effectively target areas of concern while promoting overall strength, mobility, and well-being. Incorporate these tailored isometric exercises into your regular routine to experience the benefits of improved mobility, enhanced balance, and increased functional capacity, allowing you to live life to the fullest with confidence and vitality.

Chapter 5
Targeting Specific Health Concerns
Isometric Exercises for Arthritis Relief and Joint Mobility

Arthritis can significantly impact joint mobility and overall quality of life, making it essential to incorporate exercises that promote relief and improve mobility. Isometric exercises offer a gentle yet effective approach to managing arthritis symptoms by strengthening the muscles around affected joints and improving stability without placing excessive stress on the joints themselves. In this section, we'll explore a series of isometric exercises specifically designed to provide relief for arthritis and enhance joint mobility.

1. Isometric Hand Grips:
- Sit comfortably in a chair with your back supported and your feet flat on the floor.
- Hold a soft ball or stress ball in one hand, placing it between your fingers and palm.
- Squeeze the ball firmly with your fingers and palm, holding the contraction for 5-10 seconds.
- Release the grip and relax your hand.
- Repeat the exercise for 10-15 repetitions on each hand, gradually increasing the hold time as tolerated.

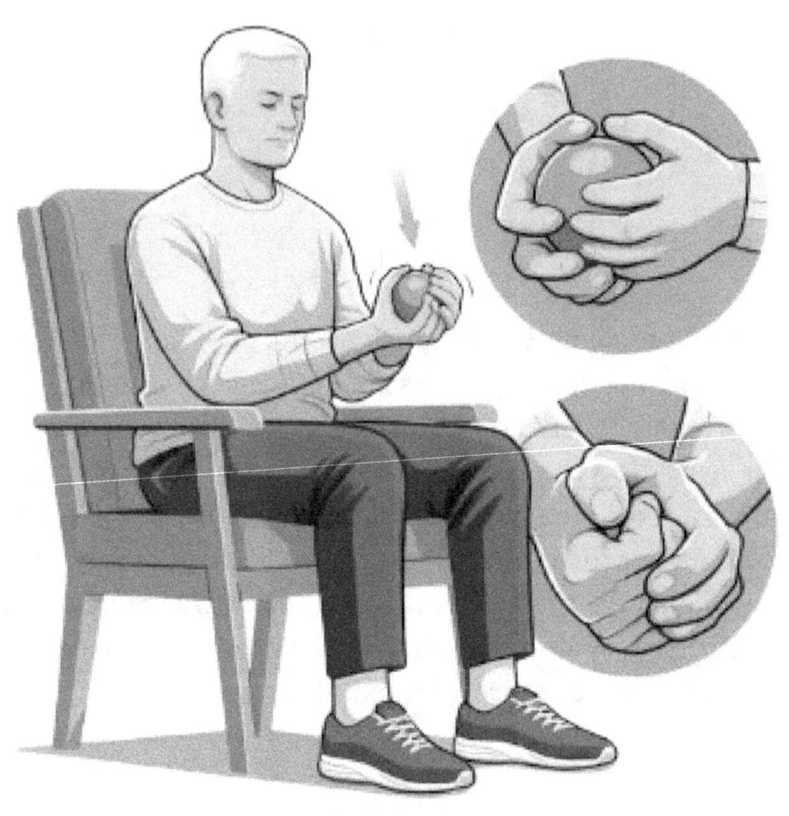

2. *Isometric Shoulder Press:*

- Sit or stand with your back straight and your shoulders relaxed.
- Hold a lightweight dumbbell or resistance band in each hand, with your elbows bent at 90 degrees and your palms facing forward.
- Press the weights or band overhead, straightening your arms while keeping your elbows at shoulder height.
- Hold the overhead position for 5-10 seconds, focusing on engaging your shoulder muscles.
- Lower the weights or band back to the starting position and repeat for 10-15 repetitions.

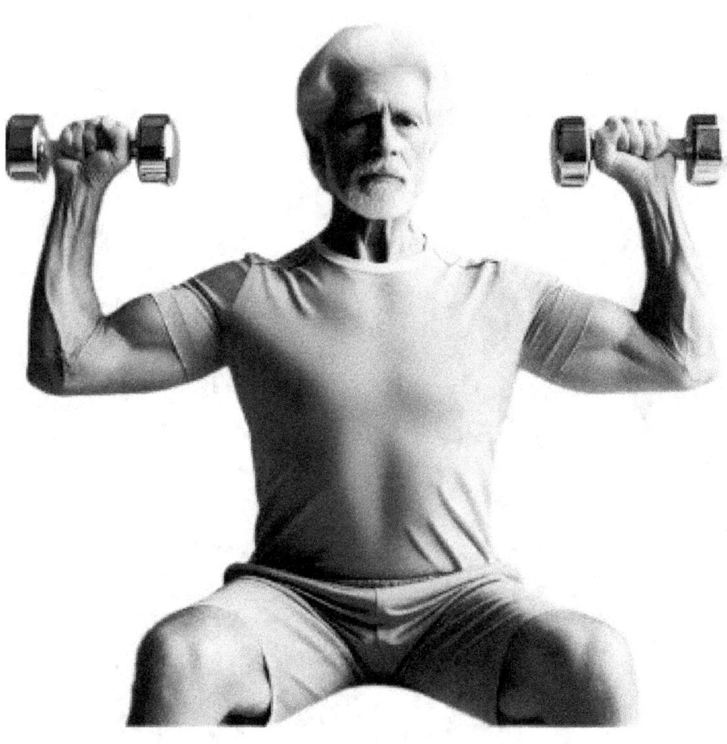

3. *Isometric Leg Press:*

- Sit in a chair with your feet flat on the floor and your knees bent at a 90-degree angle.
- Place a rolled towel or small cushion between your knees.
- Press your knees together, squeezing the towel or cushion firmly, and hold the contraction for 5-10 seconds.
- Relax and release the pressure, allowing the towel or cushion to return to its original position.
- Repeat the exercise for 10-15 repetitions, focusing on maintaining proper alignment and engaging your leg muscles.

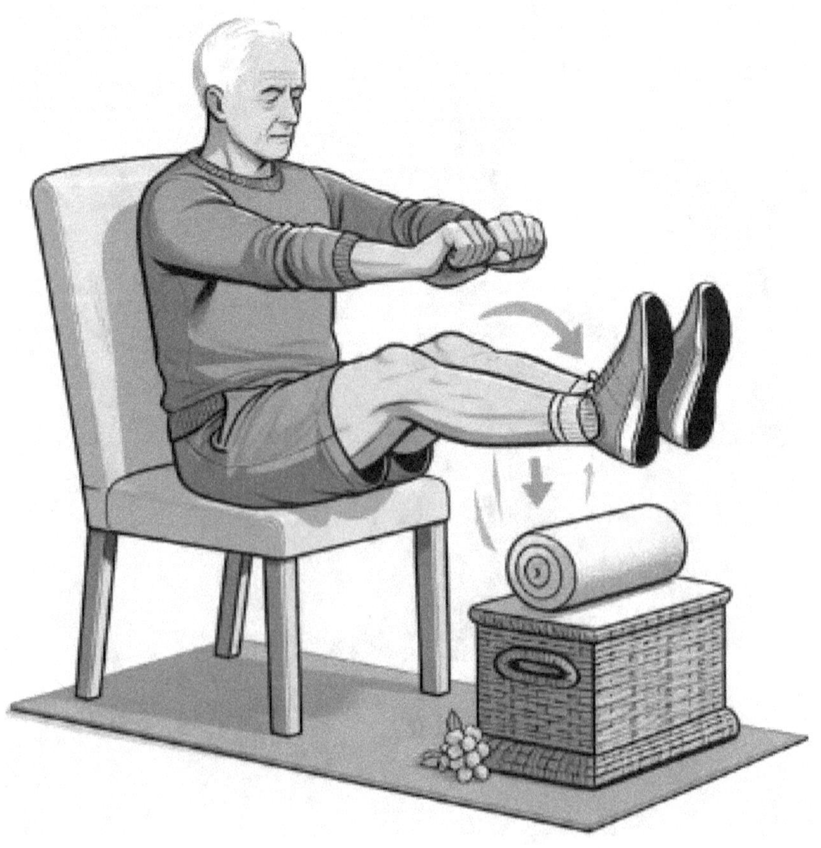

4. *Isometric Calf Raise:*

- Stand with your feet hip-width apart and your hands resting on a stable surface for support.
- Lift your heels off the ground, rising onto the balls of your feet.
- Hold the raised position for 5-10 seconds, focusing on engaging your calf muscles.
- Lower your heels back to the ground and repeat for 10-15 repetitions, maintaining balance and stability throughout.

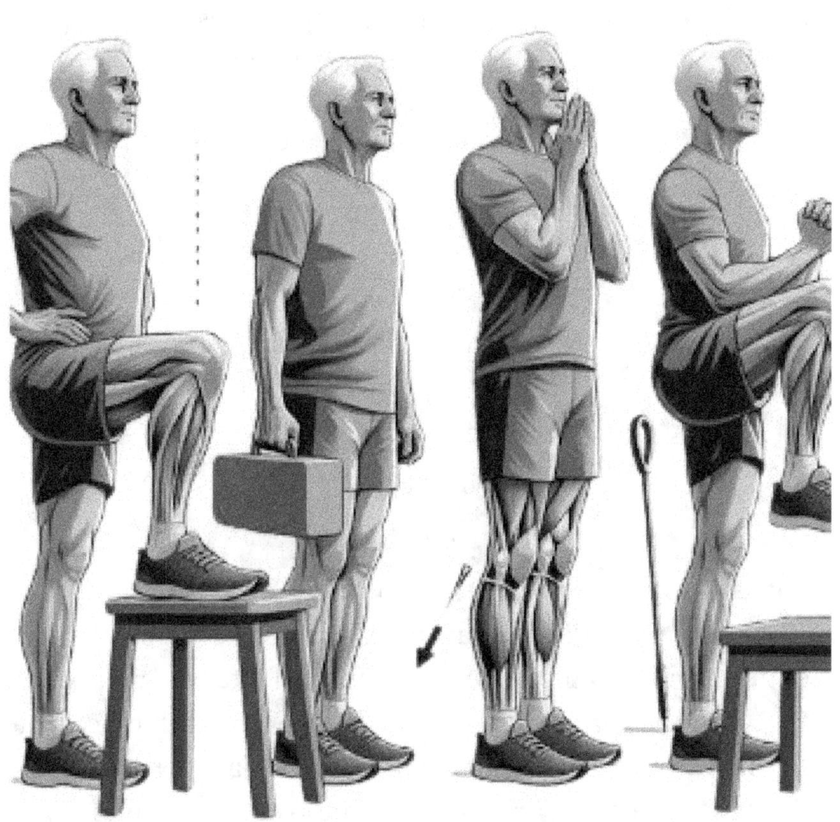

5. Isometric Chest Press:

- Sit or stand with your back straight and your shoulders relaxed.
- Hold a resistance band or towel at chest height, with your elbows bent and your palms facing forward.
- Press outward against the resistance of the band or towel, engaging your chest muscles.
- Hold the outward position for 5-10 seconds, feeling the tension in your chest.
- Relax and release the pressure, allowing the band or towel to return to its starting position.
- Repeat the exercise for 10-15 repetitions, focusing on controlled movements and proper breathing.

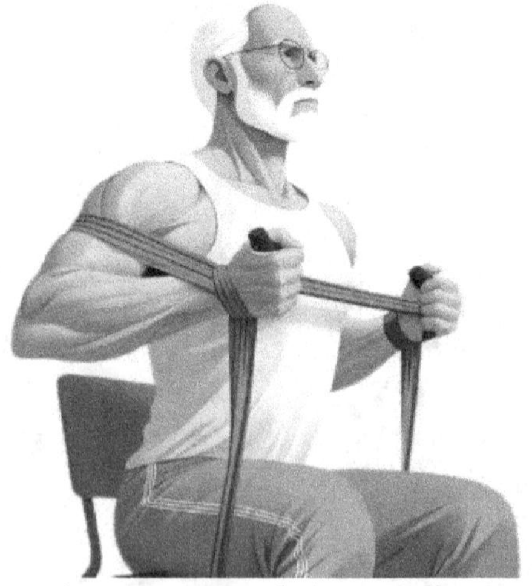

Incorporating these targeted isometric exercises into your routine can help alleviate arthritis symptoms, improve joint mobility, and enhance overall quality of life. Remember to start gradually and listen to your body, adjusting the intensity and duration of each exercise as needed. With consistent practice and dedication, you can effectively manage arthritis and enjoy greater comfort, mobility, and freedom of movement.

Strengthening Bones: Isometric Strategies for Osteoporosis Management

Osteoporosis is a condition characterized by weakened bones, making individuals more susceptible to fractures and breaks. However, incorporating isometric exercises into your routine can help strengthen bones, improve bone density, and manage osteoporosis effectively. In this section, we'll explore a series of isometric strategies specifically designed to promote bone health and enhance osteoporosis management.

1. Wall Sit with Calf Raises:

- Stand with your back against a sturdy wall and your feet hip-width apart.
- Lower yourself into a wall sit position, bending your knees to a 90-degree angle and pressing your lower back into the wall.
- Hold the wall sit position and simultaneously lift your heels off the ground, rising onto the balls of your feet.
- Hold the calf raise position for 5-10 seconds, feeling the tension in your calf muscles.
- Lower your heels back to the ground and repeat for 10-15 repetitions, focusing on controlled movements and maintaining proper form.

- Lie on your back with your knees bent and your feet flat on the floor.
- Place your hands behind your head, elbows pointing outward.
- Lift your head, neck, and shoulders slightly off the floor, engaging your abdominal muscles.
- Extend one leg straight out in front of you, hovering above the floor.
- Hold the isometric contraction for 5-10 seconds, feeling the tension in your abdominal muscles.
- Return your leg to the starting position and repeat on the opposite side.
- Aim for 10-15 repetitions on each leg, focusing on controlled movements and maintaining core stability.

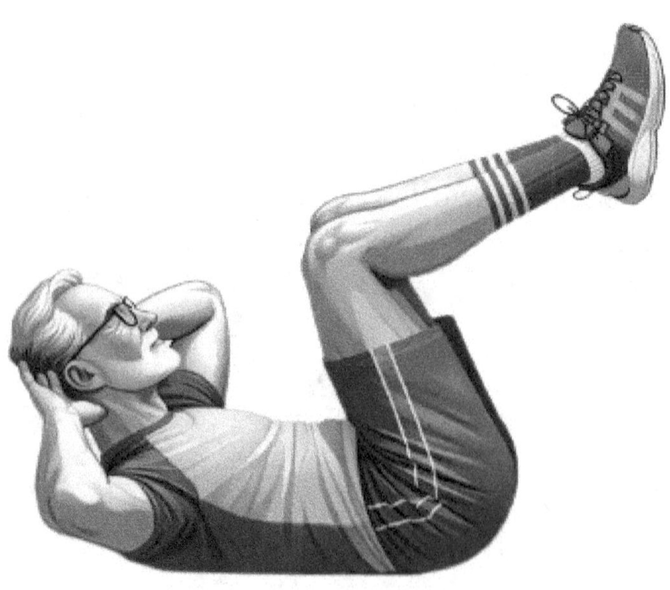

3. *Isometric Squat Hold:*

- Stand with your feet shoulder-width apart and your arms at your sides.
- Lower yourself into a squat position, bending your knees and lowering your hips as if sitting back into a chair.
- Hold the squat position for 10-20 seconds, focusing on maintaining tension in your leg muscles.
- Keep your chest lifted, shoulders back, and knees aligned with your ankles.
- Rise back up to standing and repeat for 3-5 repetitions, gradually increasing the hold time as tolerated.

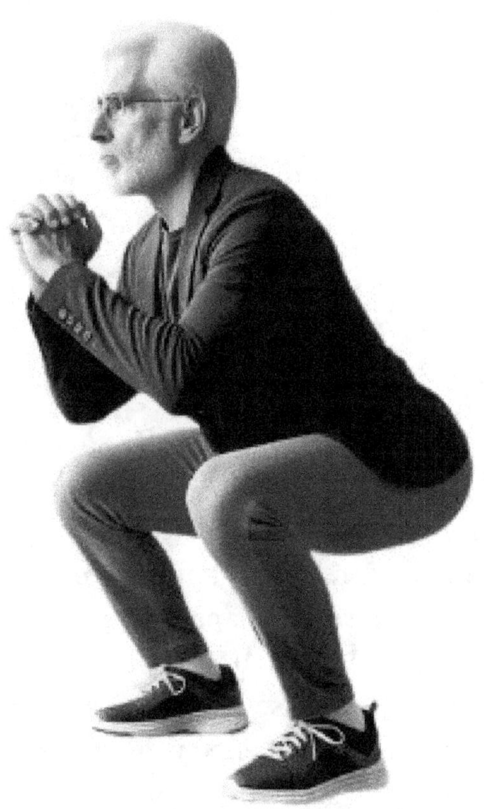

4. Isometric Hip Bridge:

- Lie on your back with your knees bent and your feet flat on the floor.
- Place your arms at your sides with your palms facing down.
- Lift your hips off the floor, engaging your glutes and hamstrings.
- Hold the bridge position for 10-20 seconds, focusing on squeezing your glutes.
- Keep your core engaged and your pelvis level throughout the exercise.
- Lower your hips back to the floor and repeat for 3-5 repetitions, focusing on controlled movements and proper breathing.

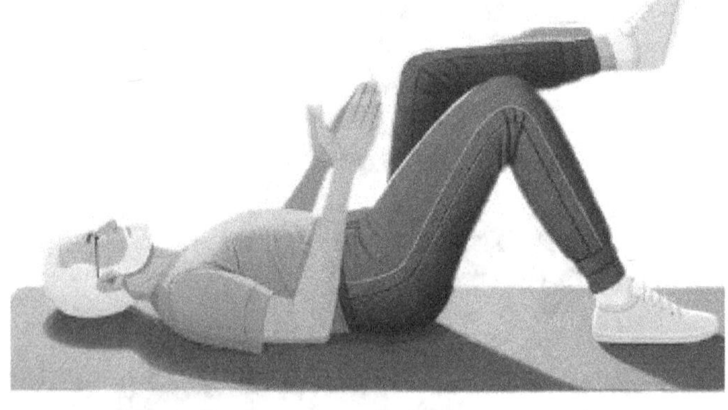

Incorporating these targeted isometric strategies into your routine can help strengthen bones, improve bone density, and enhance osteoporosis management. Remember to start gradually and listen to your body, adjusting the intensity and duration of each exercise as needed. With consistent practice and dedication, you can effectively manage osteoporosis and enjoy greater bone strength, stability, and overall well-being.

Enhancing Balance and Coordination Through Targeted Workouts

Balance and coordination are essential components of functional movement and overall well-being, particularly as we age. Targeted workouts focused on enhancing balance and coordination can help improve stability, reduce the risk of falls, and enhance overall mobility and confidence. In this section, we'll explore a series of exercises specifically designed to enhance balance and coordination through targeted workouts.

1. Single-Leg Balance:

- Stand tall with your feet hip-width apart and your arms at your sides.
- Lift one foot off the ground and balance on the opposite leg.
- Engage your core muscles and focus on maintaining your balance for 20-30 seconds.
- Keep your standing leg slightly bent and your gaze fixed on a stationary object for stability.
- Switch legs and repeat the exercise for 3-5 repetitions on each side, gradually increasing the hold time as your balance improves.

2. Toe Taps:

- Stand behind a stable surface such as a chair or countertop for support.
- Lift one foot slightly off the ground and tap your toe lightly in front of you.
- Return your foot to the starting position and tap it out to the side.
- Alternate between tapping your toe in front of you and out to the side for 10-15 repetitions on each leg.
- Focus on maintaining stability through your standing leg and controlling the movement of your tapping foot.

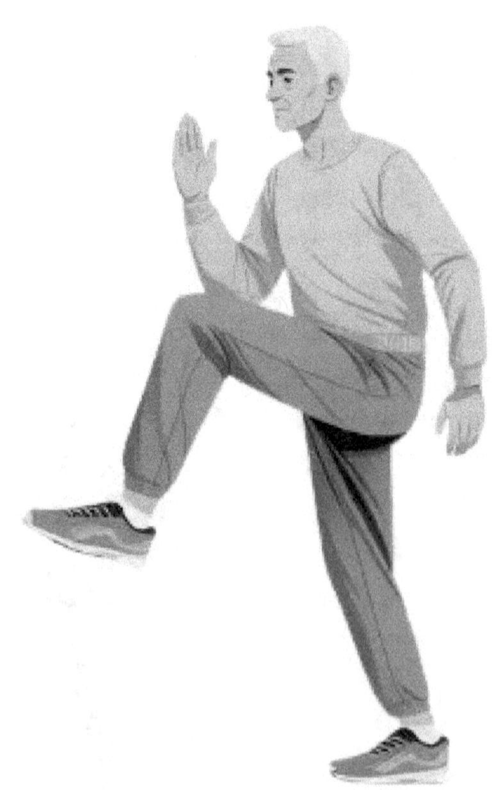

3. Tandem Stance:

- Stand with your feet together and your arms at your sides.
- Take a step forward with one foot, placing it directly in front of the other foot.
- Maintain a narrow stance with your heel of the front foot touching the toes of the back foot.
- Hold the tandem stance for 20-30 seconds, focusing on keeping your body aligned and your core engaged.
- Switch legs and repeat the exercise for 3-5 repetitions on each side, gradually increasing the hold time as your balance improves.

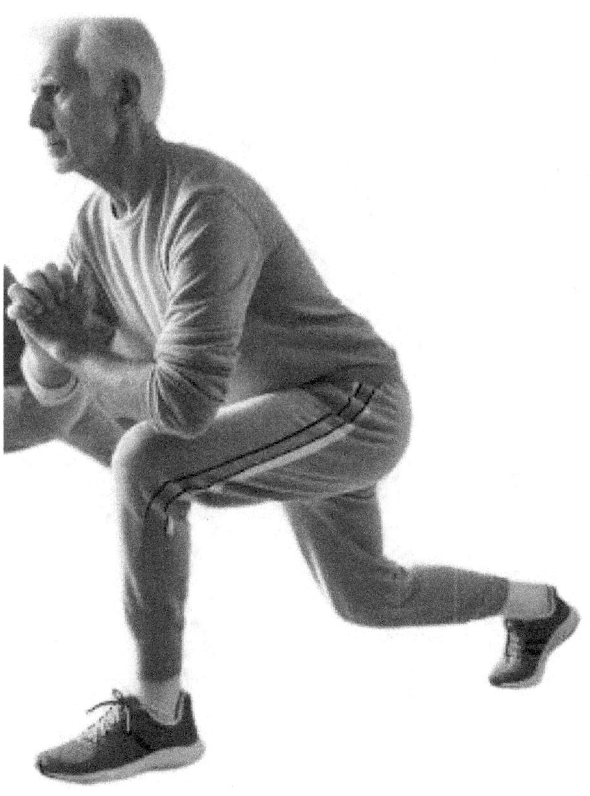

4. Heel-to-Toe Walk:

- Begin by standing with your feet together and your arms at your sides.
- Take a step forward with one foot, placing the heel of that foot directly in front of the toes of the opposite foot.
- Continue walking in a straight line, placing each foot directly in front of the other in a heel-to-toe fashion.
- Focus on maintaining a steady pace and keeping your gaze fixed on a point in front of you for balance.
- Walk for 10-15 steps forward, then reverse direction and walk back to the starting point.

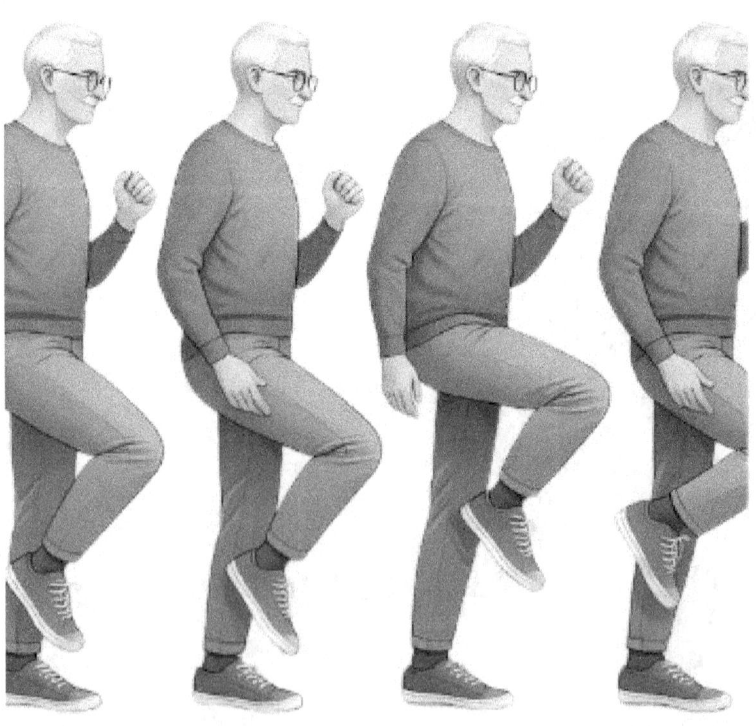

- Stand tall with your feet hip-width apart and your arms at your sides.
- Lift one foot slightly off the ground and balance on the opposite leg.
- Slowly raise your arms out to the sides and overhead, forming a "Y" shape with your body.
- Hold the balance position with your arms raised for 10-15 seconds, focusing on maintaining stability and control.
- Lower your arms and return to the starting position, then switch legs and repeat the exercise on the opposite side.

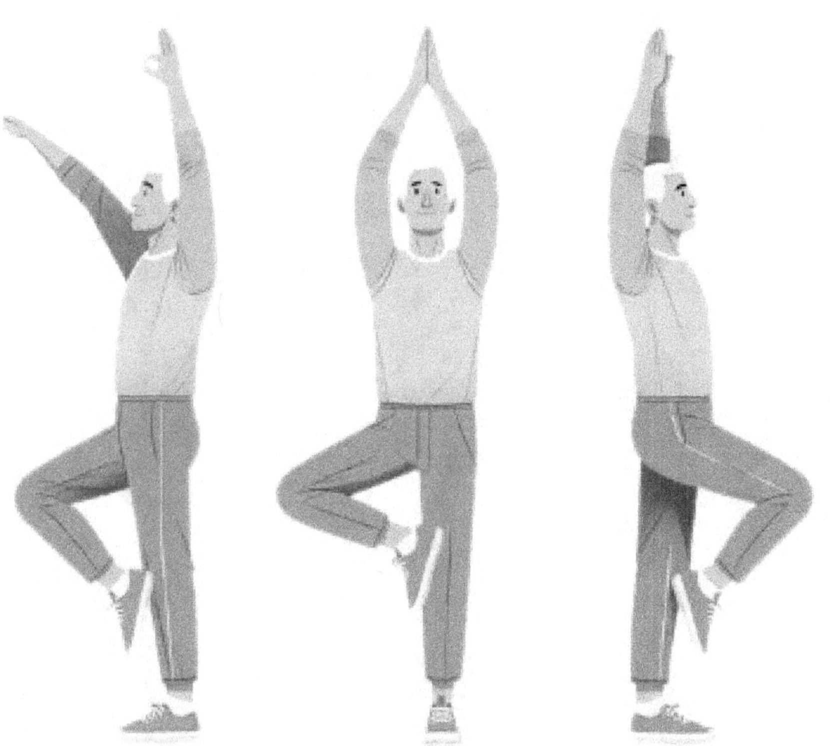

Incorporating these targeted exercises into your routine can help enhance balance and coordination, reducing the risk of falls and improving overall mobility and confidence. Start gradually and progress at your own pace, focusing on proper form and control throughout each exercise. With consistent practice and dedication, you can enjoy the benefits of improved balance and coordination, allowing you to move with greater ease and grace in your daily activities.

Chapter 6
Beyond the Physical: Nurturing Mental Well-Being
Harnessing the Psychological Benefits of Isometric Training

In the realm of fitness and exercise, the focus often tends to be primarily on the physical benefits. However, it's important to recognize that nurturing mental well-being is equally essential for overall health and vitality. Isometric training not only strengthens the body but also offers a multitude of psychological benefits that contribute to mental well-being. In this section, we'll explore how isometric training can harness these psychological benefits and support mental health.

1. Stress Reduction:

Isometric training provides an opportunity to focus solely on the present moment, shifting attention away from stressors and worries. Engaging in isometric exercises promotes relaxation and reduces tension in the body, helping to alleviate stress and promote a sense of calm and well-being.

2. Mindfulness and Meditation:

Isometric exercises require concentration and focus, akin to mindfulness and meditation practices. By tuning into the sensations of muscle engagement and breath, individuals can cultivate a greater awareness of their bodies and minds, fostering a deeper connection and presence in the moment.

3. Mood Enhancement:

Physical activity, including isometric training, triggers the release of endorphins, chemicals in the brain that act as natural mood lifters. Regular engagement in isometric exercises can help alleviate symptoms of depression and anxiety, promoting a more positive outlook and enhanced emotional well-being.

4. Confidence Building:

As individuals progress in their isometric training journey and witness improvements in strength, stability, and endurance, they often experience a boost in self-confidence. Accomplishing new milestones and overcoming challenges fosters a sense of achievement and empowerment, contributing to greater self-esteem and self-efficacy.

5. Stress Relief and Relaxation:

Isometric exercises promote relaxation by engaging the parasympathetic nervous system, which counteracts the body's stress response. Incorporating isometric training into your routine can help reduce feelings of anxiety and tension, promoting a greater sense of calm and relaxation.

6. Cognitive Benefits:

Physical activity, including isometric training, has been shown to enhance cognitive function and protect against age-related cognitive decline. Regular engagement in isometric exercises can improve memory, attention, and executive function, sharpening mental acuity and promoting brain health.

Incorporating isometric training into your routine not only strengthens the body but also nurtures mental well-being, providing a holistic approach to health and vitality. By harnessing the psychological benefits of isometric training, individuals can cultivate greater resilience, peace of mind, and overall happiness, supporting their journey towards optimal wellness and fulfillment.

Cultivating Resilience and Confidence in Aging

As we age, it's common to face a variety of physical and emotional challenges that can impact our confidence and sense of resilience. However, with the right mindset and approach, it's possible to cultivate resilience and confidence, enabling us to navigate the aging process with grace and positivity. In this section, we'll explore strategies for fostering resilience and confidence in aging, empowering individuals to embrace the opportunities and experiences that come with growing older.

1. Embracing Change:

One of the keys to cultivating resilience in aging is to embrace change as a natural part of life. Recognize that change is inevitable and that each stage of life brings new opportunities for growth and self-discovery. By adopting a mindset of acceptance and adaptability, individuals can navigate transitions with greater ease and resilience.

2. Maintaining a Positive Outlook:

Cultivating confidence in aging begins with maintaining a positive outlook on life. Focus on the aspects of aging that bring joy, fulfillment, and wisdom. Practice gratitude for the experiences and relationships that enrich your life, and approach each day with optimism and enthusiasm for what lies ahead.

3. Prioritizing Self-Care:

Taking care of oneself is essential for fostering resilience and confidence in aging. Prioritize self-care activities that nourish your body, mind, and spirit, such as regular exercise, healthy eating, adequate sleep, and relaxation techniques. Investing in your well-being empowers you to face life's challenges with strength and vitality.

4. Setting Realistic Goals:

Setting realistic goals and aspirations can boost confidence and provide a sense of purpose in aging. Identify areas of interest or passion and set achievable goals that align with your values and priorities. Celebrate your accomplishments along the way, no matter how small, and use setbacks as opportunities for growth and learning.

5. Cultivating Social Connections:

Maintaining strong social connections is vital for resilience and confidence in aging. Nurture relationships with family, friends, and community members who uplift and support you. Seek out opportunities for social engagement and meaningful connections, whether through volunteering, joining clubs or groups, or participating in social activities.

6. Embracing Lifelong Learning:

Continuing to learn and grow throughout life fosters resilience and confidence in aging. Stay curious and open-minded, exploring new interests, hobbies, and experiences. Engage in lifelong learning opportunities such as classes, workshops, or online courses that stimulate your mind and expand your horizons.

Finally, don't hesitate to seek support when needed. Reach out to trusted friends, family members, or professionals for guidance, encouragement, and assistance. Asking for help is a sign of strength, and receiving support can provide valuable resources and perspectives to help you navigate challenges with resilience and confidence.

By embracing change, maintaining a positive outlook, prioritizing self-care, setting realistic goals, cultivating social connections, embracing lifelong learning, and seeking support, individuals can cultivate resilience and confidence in aging. With these strategies in place, aging becomes not just a process of growing older but an opportunity for personal growth, fulfillment, and empowerment.

Chapter 7
Incorporating Isometric Workouts into Daily Life
Integrating Isometric Exercises into Your Regular Routine

Isometric exercises offer a convenient and effective way to improve strength, flexibility, and overall fitness without the need for specialized equipment or dedicated workout sessions. By integrating isometric exercises into your daily routine, you can reap the benefits of these exercises without disrupting your schedule. In this section, we'll explore strategies for seamlessly incorporating isometric workouts into your daily life.

1. Morning Routine:

Start your day with a few minutes of isometric exercises to energize your body and prepare for the day ahead. Consider incorporating isometric squats, wall push-ups, or plank holds into your morning routine while brushing your teeth or waiting for your coffee to brew.

2. Work Breaks:

Take short breaks throughout your workday to perform quick isometric exercises that can be done at your desk or in your workspace. Stand up and do calf raises, chair squats, or shoulder presses using resistance bands. These exercises can help combat the effects of sitting for long periods and boost your energy levels.

3. Household Chores:

Turn household chores into opportunities for physical activity by incorporating isometric exercises into your cleaning routine. While washing dishes, waiting for laundry, or vacuuming, engage your muscles with wall sits, countertop push-ups, or holding a squat position while folding clothes.

4. Commute or Travel Time:

If you commute to work or spend time traveling, use this time to sneak in some isometric exercises. While sitting on public transportation or waiting at the airport, perform seated leg lifts, abdominal contractions, or calf raises. These exercises can help pass the time and keep your muscles engaged.

5. TV Time:

Instead of being sedentary while watching TV or streaming your favorite shows, incorporate isometric exercises into your viewing routine. Perform wall sits, glute bridges, or static lunges during commercial breaks or while binge-watching your favorite series. You'll maximize your leisure time while improving your fitness.

6. Evening Wind Down:

Wind down in the evening with a relaxing routine that includes gentle isometric stretches and exercises. Perform seated forward bends, chest stretches against a wall, or overhead reaches while winding down before bed. These exercises can help release tension built up during the day and promote relaxation for a restful sleep.

By integrating isometric exercises into your daily routine, you can make fitness a natural and effortless part of your lifestyle. Whether you're at home, at work, or on the go, there are plenty of opportunities to incorporate these exercises into your day without adding extra time or complexity. With consistency and commitment, you'll experience the benefits of improved strength, flexibility, and overall well-being.

Overcoming Challenges and Maintaining Consistency

Embarking on a fitness journey, including incorporating isometric workouts into your routine, often comes with its fair share of challenges. From time constraints to lack of motivation, overcoming obstacles is essential for maintaining consistency and achieving long-term success. In this section, we'll explore strategies for overcoming challenges and maintaining consistency in your isometric workout regimen.

1. Identify Potential Obstacles:

The first step in overcoming challenges is to identify the obstacles that may hinder your consistency. Whether it's a busy schedule, lack of energy, or competing priorities, pinpointing the barriers to your workouts allows you to develop strategies to overcome them effectively.

2. Set Realistic Goals:

Establishing clear, achievable goals can help you stay motivated and focused on your fitness journey. Break down your long-term objectives into smaller, manageable milestones, and celebrate each achievement along the way. By setting realistic goals, you'll maintain momentum and keep moving forward, even when faced with challenges.

3. Prioritize Self-Care:

Taking care of your physical and mental well-being is crucial for maintaining consistency in your workouts. Make self-care a priority by getting enough sleep, eating a balanced diet, managing stress, and practicing relaxation techniques. When you feel your best, you're more likely to stay committed to your fitness routine. **64**

4. Create a Supportive Environment:

Surround yourself with a supportive network of friends, family, or workout buddies who encourage and motivate you on your fitness journey. Share your goals and challenges with others, and lean on them for support when needed. A supportive environment can help you stay accountable and inspired to keep pushing forward.

5. Be Flexible and Adapt:

Flexibility is key to overcoming challenges and maintaining consistency in your workouts. Be willing to adapt your exercise routine based on changing circumstances, such as unexpected events or time constraints. Explore alternative workout options, such as shorter workouts or at-home routines, to ensure you can stay on track no matter what life throws your way.

6. Focus on the Benefits:

Remind yourself of the numerous benefits of regular exercise, including improved physical health, mental well-being, and overall quality of life. Keep your eyes on the prize and stay focused on the positive outcomes of your efforts. Visualize yourself achieving your goals and imagine how you'll feel when you reach them.

7. Practice Self-Compassion:

It's important to be kind to yourself and practice self-compassion, especially during challenging times. If you miss a workout or encounter setbacks, don't be too hard on yourself. Instead, acknowledge your efforts and focus on moving forward with renewed determination and resilience.

8. Stay Consistent:

Consistency is key to long-term success in any fitness regimen. Make a commitment to yourself to prioritize your workouts and stick to your plan, even when faced with challenges. Remember that every small step you take towards your goals contributes to your overall progress and success.

By implementing these strategies, you can overcome challenges and maintain consistency in your isometric workout routine. With perseverance, determination, and a positive mindset, you'll overcome obstacles and achieve your fitness goals, paving the way for a healthier, happier, and more fulfilling life.

Chapter 8
Realizing the Rewards: Transforming Your Life Through Isometric Workouts
Celebrating Success Stories and Personal Achievements

Isometric workouts have the power to transform not only your physical fitness but also your overall well-being and quality of life. In this section, we'll explore the rewards of incorporating isometric exercises into your routine and celebrate the success stories and personal achievements that come with embracing this fitness approach.

1. Improved Physical Health:

By engaging in regular isometric workouts, you can experience a wide range of physical health benefits. Strengthening your muscles, improving flexibility, and enhancing overall fitness contribute to better posture, reduced risk of injury, and increased longevity. Celebrate the improvements in your physical health as you feel stronger, more energetic, and capable of taking on daily challenges with ease.

2. Enhanced Mental Well-Being:

Isometric workouts not only strengthen the body but also support mental well-being. The release of endorphins during exercise can uplift your mood, reduce stress, and alleviate symptoms of anxiety and depression.

Take pride in the mental clarity, emotional resilience, and inner peace that come from prioritizing your fitness and self-care.

3. Increased Confidence and Self-Esteem:

As you progress in your isometric training journey and witness improvements in strength, endurance, and physical appearance, you'll likely experience a boost in confidence and self-esteem. Celebrate the newfound sense of empowerment and self-assurance that comes from achieving your fitness goals and overcoming challenges along the way.

4. Greater Sense of Achievement:

Each milestone reached and personal achievement unlocked through your isometric workouts is worth celebrating. Whether it's mastering a challenging exercise, surpassing a personal best, or consistently sticking to your workout routine, acknowledge and celebrate your accomplishments as markers of your dedication and determination.

5. Enhanced Quality of Life:

Embracing isometric workouts can lead to a significant enhancement in your overall quality of life. Enjoy the increased energy levels, improved sleep quality, and greater vitality that accompany regular exercise. Celebrate the newfound sense of freedom and fulfillment that comes from living a healthier, more active lifestyle.

6. Inspirational Success Stories:

Take inspiration from the success stories of others who have transformed their lives through isometric workouts.

Whether it's overcoming physical limitations, achieving remarkable fitness milestones, or reclaiming their health and vitality, these stories serve as powerful reminders of the transformative power of exercise and determination.

7. Personal Achievements:

Reflect on your own personal achievements and milestones in your isometric training journey. Whether it's completing a challenging workout program, reaching a weight loss goal, or experiencing improvements in strength and mobility, each achievement is a testament to your dedication and perseverance.

By realizing the rewards of isometric workouts and celebrating success stories and personal achievements, you can fully appreciate the transformative impact that fitness can have on your life. Embrace the journey, acknowledge your progress, and take pride in the positive changes you've made for your health and well-being. With each workout, you're one step closer to becoming the best version of yourself.

Embracing a Future Filled with Vitality, Wellness, and Possibility

As we embark on our journey towards better health and well-being through isometric workouts, it's important to envision a future brimming with vitality, wellness, and endless possibilities. In this section, we'll explore the transformative potential of embracing a lifestyle centered around fitness and self-care, and the boundless opportunities it brings for a fulfilling and vibrant future.

1. Embracing Vitality:

By prioritizing regular isometric workouts and adopting healthy lifestyle habits, we can revitalize our bodies and cultivate a deep sense of vitality. Imagine waking up each day feeling energized, resilient, and ready to tackle whatever challenges come your way. Embracing vitality means embracing life to the fullest, with boundless energy and enthusiasm for each new day.

2. Pursuing Wellness:

Wellness encompasses not only physical health but also mental, emotional, and spiritual well-being. Through isometric workouts, mindfulness practices, and self-care rituals, we can nurture holistic wellness and create a life of balance and harmony. Picture yourself thriving in all areas of your life – physically strong, mentally resilient, emotionally fulfilled, and spiritually grounded.

3. Seizing Opportunities:

As we commit to our fitness journey and prioritize our health, we open ourselves up to a world of possibilities and opportunities.

Imagine the doors that will open when you're feeling your best, new career opportunities, exciting adventures, meaningful relationships, and personal growth experiences await. By embracing fitness and well-being, we empower ourselves to seize every opportunity that comes our way.

4. Embracing Aging with Grace:

Aging is a natural part of life, and by embracing fitness and wellness, we can navigate the aging process with grace and dignity. Picture yourself aging gracefully, with strength, vitality, and wisdom. Embrace each new chapter of life with confidence and resilience, knowing that you've laid the foundation for a vibrant and fulfilling future through your commitment to health and fitness.

5. Inspiring Others:

By leading by example and prioritizing your health and well-being, you have the power to inspire others to do the same. Imagine the ripple effect of your actions – friends, family members, and even strangers inspired to embark on their own fitness journey and transform their lives for the better. Your commitment to vitality and wellness has the potential to create a ripple effect of positive change in the world.

6. Creating a Legacy of Health:

As you embrace a future filled with vitality, wellness, and possibility, you're not only transforming your own life but also creating a legacy of health for future generations. Imagine the impact of passing down a legacy of health and well-being to your children, grandchildren, and beyond. By prioritizing fitness and self-care, you're setting a powerful example for generations to come.

By embracing a future filled with vitality, wellness, and possibility, we unlock the true potential of our lives and create a legacy of health and happiness that extends far beyond ourselves. Through isometric workouts and a commitment to self-care, we can shape a future brimming with vitality, wellness, and endless opportunities for growth, fulfillment, and joy.

Conclusion

In conclusion, "Isometric Workouts for Older Adults: Unlocking Vitality and Wellness After 50 with Tailored Exercises for Age-Related Challenges" serves as a comprehensive guide to achieving optimal health and well-being through the power of isometric exercises. Throughout this journey, we've explored the science behind isometric training, learned essential techniques, addressed common age-related conditions, and discovered strategies for overcoming challenges and maintaining consistency.

By embracing isometric workouts, individuals can transform their lives, cultivating strength, resilience, and confidence as they age. The benefits extend beyond the physical, encompassing mental, emotional, and spiritual wellness. With dedication, perseverance, and a positive mindset, readers can embark on a path towards a future filled with vitality, wellness, and endless possibilities.

As we close this chapter, let us carry forward the lessons learned and the inspiration gained from these pages. Let us continue to prioritize our health, embrace the journey of aging with grace and resilience, and inspire others to do the same. With each step we take towards better health and well-being, we move closer to realizing our full potential and creating a legacy of vitality and wellness for generations to come.

Thank you for joining us on this transformative journey. May your path be filled with strength, vitality, and abundant wellness as you continue to thrive in the years ahead.